THE COMPLETE 2024 DIVERTICULITIS DIET COOKBOOK

100+ Flavorful Recipes to Rejuvenate Your Gut Health and Essential Guidance for Diverticulitis Management

LUCKY WILSON

Copyright © 2024 by Lucky Wilson

Table of Contents

INTRODUCTION

Understanding Diverticulitis

Diverticulitis is a condition characterized by the inflammation or infection of small, bulging pouches called diverticula that can form in the lining of the digestive system. These pouches are most commonly found in the lower part of the large intestine (colon). Diverticulitis can cause severe abdominal pain, fever, nausea, and a marked change in bowel habits. Understanding this condition involves delving into its causes, symptoms, diagnosis, treatment, and preventive measures.

Causes of Diverticulitis

The exact cause of diverticulitis is not completely understood, but it is generally believed to be associated with the formation of diverticula. These pouches can develop when naturally weak places in the colon give way under pressure, causing marble-sized pouches to protrude through the colon wall. Several factors contribute to this process:

1. Diet: A low-fiber diet is often cited as a significant factor. Fiber helps soften stool and prevent constipation, which reduces pressure in the colon. Diets low in fiber can lead to harder stools and increased colon pressure, contributing to the formation of diverticula.
2. Age: The risk of developing diverticula and consequently diverticulitis increases with age, particularly after the age of 40.
3. Genetics: A family history of diverticulitis may increase an individual's risk.
4. Lifestyle Factors: Lack of physical activity, obesity, and smoking have all been linked to an increased risk of diverticulitis.

Symptoms of Diverticulitis

Diverticulitis can present a range of symptoms, from mild to severe. Common symptoms include:

1. Abdominal Pain: Typically in the lower left side, though it can occur on the right side as well.
2. Fever and Chills: Often indicative of an infection.
3. Nausea and Vomiting: These symptoms can accompany abdominal pain.
4. Changes in Bowel Habits: These might include constipation, diarrhea, or a combination of both.
5. Bloating and Gas: Discomfort and bloating are common, especially after meals.
6. Loss of Appetite: Due to pain and nausea, individuals may find eating difficult.

Diagnosis of Diverticulitis

Diagnosing diverticulitis typically involves a combination of medical history, physical examination, and diagnostic tests:

1. Medical History and Physical Exam: The doctor will review symptoms and medical history and

perform a physical exam, particularly focusing on the abdomen.

2. Blood Tests: These can help detect signs of infection, such as an elevated white blood cell count.

3. Imaging Tests: A CT scan is the most common and effective way to diagnose diverticulitis, revealing inflamed or infected diverticula.

4. Stool Tests: These may be used to rule out other conditions, such as infections or inflammatory bowel diseases.

Treatment of Diverticulitis

Treatment for diverticulitis depends on the severity of the condition:

1. Mild Cases: Often treated with rest, dietary modifications, and antibiotics. A clear liquid diet may be recommended initially to allow the colon to heal, gradually progressing to a low-fiber diet.

2. Moderate to Severe Cases: These may require hospitalization. Treatment can include intravenous antibiotics, pain management, and sometimes surgery if complications arise, such as abscesses, perforation, or bowel obstruction.

3. Surgical Intervention: In cases of recurrent diverticulitis or complications, surgery may be necessary to remove the affected portion of the colon.

Prevention of Diverticulitis

Preventing diverticulitis largely focuses on dietary and lifestyle changes to reduce the formation of diverticula and prevent inflammation:

1. High-Fiber Diet: Consuming a diet rich in fiber (fruits, vegetables, whole grains, and legumes) helps maintain regular bowel movements and reduce colon pressure.

2. Hydration: Drinking plenty of fluids helps keep stools soft and prevents constipation.

3. Regular Exercise: Physical activity promotes regular bowel movements and overall digestive health.

4. Weight Management: Maintaining a healthy weight reduces the risk of diverticulitis.

5. Avoid Smoking: Smoking cessation can lower the risk of diverticulitis and other gastrointestinal issues.

Living with Diverticulitis

Managing diverticulitis involves being mindful of dietary choices, staying hydrated, and leading an active lifestyle. Individuals should work closely with their healthcare providers to monitor their condition and make necessary adjustments to their treatment plan. Regular check-ups and open communication with medical professionals are crucial for effective management and prevention of complications.

Importance of Diet in Diverticulitis Management

Diverticulitis, an inflammation or infection of small pouches (diverticula) that can form in the walls of the colon, requires comprehensive management to prevent recurrence and complications. Among the various aspects of managing diverticulitis, diet plays a pivotal role. Proper dietary habits can help manage symptoms during acute episodes, facilitate recovery, and prevent future flare-ups. Understanding the importance of diet in diverticulitis management involves exploring the types of foods to eat and avoid, the role of fiber, and practical dietary strategies.

Role of Fiber in Diverticulitis Management

Dietary fiber is crucial in managing diverticulitis, primarily because it helps regulate bowel movements and reduce pressure in the colon. There are two main types of fiber:

1. Soluble Fiber: Found in foods like oats, beans, and certain fruits, soluble fiber dissolves in water to

form a gel-like substance. This type of fiber helps lower cholesterol and blood sugar levels.

2. Insoluble Fiber: Found in whole grains, nuts, and vegetables, insoluble fiber adds bulk to stool and aids in its passage through the digestive tract. For individuals with diverticulitis, a high-fiber diet is generally recommended to help prevent the formation of diverticula and reduce the risk of inflammation. Fiber softens stool, making it easier to pass and decreasing the likelihood of constipation, which can contribute to the formation of diverticula by increasing pressure in the colon.

Diet During Acute Diverticulitis Flare-Ups

During an acute diverticulitis episode, the primary goal is to allow the colon to rest and heal. Dietary modifications are crucial during this period:

1. Clear Liquid Diet: Initially, a clear liquid diet may be recommended. This includes broths, clear juices,

gelatin, and water. A clear liquid diet helps maintain hydration while minimizing bowel activity.

2. Low-Fiber Diet: As symptoms improve, a low-fiber diet is gradually introduced. Foods like white rice, white bread, and cooked fruits and vegetables (without skins or seeds) are easier to digest and less likely to irritate the colon.

Transition to a High-Fiber Diet

Once the acute phase has resolved, transitioning to a high-fiber diet is essential for long-term management and prevention of future episodes. Key dietary strategies include:

1. Gradual Fiber Increase: Increase fiber intake gradually to allow the digestive system to adjust. Sudden increases can cause gas and bloating.

2. Variety of Fiber Sources: Incorporate a variety of high-fiber foods such as fruits (apples, pears, berries), vegetables (broccoli, carrots, leafy greens),

legumes (lentils, beans), and whole grains (brown rice, oatmeal).

3. Hydration: Adequate water intake is essential when increasing fiber consumption to help fiber move smoothly through the digestive tract and prevent constipation.

Foods to Avoid

Certain foods can aggravate diverticulitis symptoms and should be limited or avoided, especially during a flare-up:

1. Red Meat: High intake of red meat, especially processed meats, has been associated with an increased risk of diverticulitis.

2. High-Fat and Fried Foods: These can be difficult to digest and may exacerbate symptoms.

3. Seeds and Nuts: Historically, it was believed that seeds and nuts could lodge in diverticula and cause inflammation, although recent research has questioned this. However, individuals may still

choose to avoid these foods if they notice they trigger symptoms.

4. Processed Foods: Foods high in refined sugars and low in fiber can contribute to constipation and should be minimized.

Probiotics and Diverticulitis

Emerging research suggests that probiotics, beneficial bacteria found in certain foods and supplements, may help in managing diverticulitis. Probiotics can promote gut health by enhancing the balance of good bacteria in the colon. Foods like yogurt, kefir, and fermented vegetables contain probiotics and can be beneficial when included as part of a balanced diet.

Practical Dietary Tips

Small, Frequent Meals: Eating smaller, more frequent meals can help manage symptoms and improve digestion.

1. Chew Thoroughly: Properly chewing food can aid digestion and reduce the burden on the digestive system.
2. Regular Meal Times: Establishing regular eating patterns can promote regular bowel movements and overall digestive health.

Consulting a Dietitian

Working with a registered dietitian can provide personalized dietary guidance tailored to individual needs and preferences. A dietitian can help create a balanced meal plan, suggest suitable fiber sources, and address any specific dietary concerns related to diverticulitis.

How to use this cookbook

Understanding the Structure

This cookbook is organized to provide you with easy access to the information and recipes you need. It is divided into several key sections:

1. Introduction to Diverticulitis: Learn about the condition, its symptoms, causes, and the role of diet in its management.
2. Dietary Guidelines: Detailed advice on what to eat and avoid, along with tips on transitioning from a low-fiber diet during flare-ups to a high-fiber diet for long-term management.
3. Essential Tools and Ingredients: A comprehensive list of kitchen tools and staple ingredients to ensure you are well-equipped to prepare the recipes.
4. Meal Plans: Structured meal plans to guide you through different phases of managing diverticulitis.

5. Recipes: A variety of breakfast, lunch, dinner, snacks, and dessert recipes specifically designed for diverticulitis management.

Navigating the Recipes

Each recipe is crafted to be both delicious and suitable for managing diverticulitis. Here's how to navigate and utilize the recipes:

1. Recipe Categories: The recipes are categorized by meal type (breakfast, lunch, dinner, etc.) and dietary phase (low-fiber, high-fiber).
2. Ingredients and Substitutions: Ingredient lists are clear and concise. Where possible, substitutions are suggested for ingredients that may not be available or suitable for your specific dietary needs.
3. Step-by-Step Instructions: Each recipe includes easy-to-follow steps to ensure successful preparation, regardless of your cooking experience.

4. Nutritional Information: Nutritional details are provided to help you make informed choices about your meals.

Tailoring to Your Needs

Every individual's experience with diverticulitis is unique, so it's important to tailor the recipes and meal plans to your specific needs and tolerances:

1. Adjusting Portions: The recipes can be scaled up or down based on your needs. Pay attention to portion sizes to avoid overeating, which can stress the digestive system.
2. Personal Preferences: Feel free to adjust recipes based on your taste preferences while keeping within the dietary guidelines provided.
3. Tracking Triggers: Keep a food diary to track any foods that may trigger symptoms. This will help you identify and avoid problematic ingredients in the future.

Practical Tips for Success

Meal Planning: Use the meal plans as a starting point. Plan your meals for the week to ensure you have all necessary ingredients and reduce the temptation to stray from your diet.

1. Preparation: Batch cooking and meal prepping can save time and ensure you always have healthy options available, especially during busy days.
2. Stay Hydrated: Drinking plenty of water is crucial, especially when increasing your fiber intake. Aim for at least eight glasses a day.
3. Mindful Eating: Take time to chew your food thoroughly and eat slowly. This aids digestion and helps prevent overeating.

Incorporating Lifestyle Changes

Diet is just one aspect of managing diverticulitis. Consider these additional lifestyle tips:

1. Regular Exercise: Incorporate regular physical activity into your routine to promote digestive health and overall well-being.

2. Stress Management: Stress can affect your digestive system. Practice relaxation techniques such as yoga, meditation, or deep-breathing exercises.

3. Regular Medical Check-ups: Stay in touch with your healthcare provider to monitor your condition and make any necessary adjustments to your management plan.

Chapter1: Getting Started

Basics of a Diverticulitis-Friendly Diet

A diverticulitis-friendly diet aims to promote digestive health, reduce inflammation, and prevent complications associated with diverticulitis. This condition involves the formation of small pouches (diverticula) in the colon, which can become inflamed or infected. Managing diverticulitis through diet involves focusing on specific food choices and dietary habits to alleviate symptoms and support overall well-being.

Emphasis on High-Fiber Foods

1. Purpose: High-fiber foods help maintain regular bowel movements and prevent constipation, which can reduce the pressure in the colon and lower the risk of diverticula formation and inflammation.
2. Sources of Fiber: Include fruits (such as berries, apples), vegetables (like broccoli, spinach), whole grains (such as oats, quinoa), legumes (beans, lentils), and nuts (like almonds, walnuts).
3. Types of Fiber: Soluble fiber (found in oats, beans) dissolves in water and forms a gel-like substance that helps soften stool. Insoluble fiber (found in whole grains, vegetables) adds bulk to stool, aiding its passage through the digestive tract.

Foods to Avoid

1. Red Meat and Processed Foods: High intake of red meat and processed foods has been associated with increased inflammation and digestive discomfort.

2. Low-Fiber Foods: White bread, white rice, and other low-fiber foods can contribute to constipation and exacerbate symptoms.

3. Seeds and Nuts: While previously restricted, recent research suggests they may not be as problematic as once thought. However, some individuals may still choose to avoid them during acute flare-ups.

Importance of Hydration

Water Intake: Adequate hydration is crucial for maintaining soft and bulky stool, which helps prevent constipation and promotes overall digestive health.

1. Fluid Sources: Besides water, herbal teas and diluted fruit juices can contribute to daily fluid intake.

Balanced Diet Approach

1. Lean Proteins: Choose lean sources of protein such as poultry, fish, and plant-based proteins like tofu and legumes.
2. Healthy Fats: Incorporate sources of healthy fats like olive oil, avocados, and nuts in moderation.
3. Moderation in Sweets and Alcohol: Limit consumption of sugary foods and beverages as well as alcoholic drinks, which can irritate the digestive system.

Meal Planning and Preparation

1. Regular Meals: Establish regular meal times and avoid skipping meals to maintain consistent digestive function.
2. Portion Control: Monitor portion sizes to avoid overeating, which can stress the digestive system.
3. Cooking Methods: Opt for cooking methods such as steaming, baking, or grilling rather than frying,

which can add unnecessary fats and irritate the digestive tract.

Foods to Avoid on a Diverticulitis Diet

Managing diverticulitis involves avoiding certain foods that can exacerbate symptoms and increase the risk of flare-ups. Here are foods to steer clear of when following a diverticulitis diet:

Red Meat and Processed Meats:

1. Reason: High in saturated fats and often difficult to digest, which can lead to inflammation and discomfort.
2. Examples: Beef, pork, sausage, bacon, and deli meats.

High-Fat Foods:

1. Reason: These foods can contribute to inflammation and digestive distress.
2. Examples: Fried foods, fatty cuts of meat, creamy sauces, and gravies.

Low-Fiber Foods:

1. Reason: Lack of fiber can lead to constipation and increase pressure in the colon, potentially worsening diverticulitis symptoms.
2. Examples: White bread, white rice, refined cereals, and pastries.

Dairy Products:

1. Reason: Some individuals with diverticulitis may be sensitive to dairy, which can cause bloating and discomfort.
2. Examples: Full-fat dairy products like whole milk, cheese, and ice cream.

Seeds and Nuts:

1. Historical Concern: While the restriction of seeds and nuts has been debated, some individuals may still avoid them during acute flare-ups due to concerns about irritating diverticula.
2. Examples: Poppy seeds, sesame seeds, and nuts with skins (like almonds and peanuts).

Spicy Foods:

1. Reason: Spicy foods can irritate the digestive tract and may trigger symptoms in some individuals.
2. Examples: Hot peppers, chili peppers, and spicy sauces.

Popcorn and Tough Skins:

1. Reason: Hard-to-digest foods like popcorn kernels and tough skins of fruits and vegetables can potentially cause irritation.

2. Examples: Popcorn, raw apples, and raw carrots.

Alcohol and Caffeine:

1. Reason: Both alcohol and caffeine can irritate the digestive system and lead to dehydration, which may worsen diverticulitis symptoms.
2. Examples: Beer, wine, coffee, and caffeinated beverages.

Sugary Foods and Beverages:

1. Reason: High sugar intake can disrupt digestive health and contribute to inflammation.
2. Examples: Sugary snacks, desserts, and sweetened beverages.

Carbonated Beverages:

1. Reason: Carbonated drinks can cause gas and bloating, potentially exacerbating discomfort.
2. Examples: Soda, sparkling water, and fizzy drinks.

Foods to Include on a Diverticulitis Diet

Managing diverticulitis involves incorporating foods that support digestive health, reduce inflammation, and prevent flare-ups. Here are nutrient-rich foods to include in a diverticulitis diet:

High-Fiber Foods:

1. Purpose: Fiber helps maintain regular bowel movements and prevent constipation, reducing pressure in the colon.
2. Examples: Whole grains (like oats, quinoa), fruits (such as berries, apples), vegetables (like spinach, broccoli), legumes (beans, lentils), and nuts (such as almonds, walnuts).

Lean Proteins:

1. Purpose: Provides essential nutrients without excess saturated fats that can aggravate symptoms.
2. Examples: Skinless poultry (like chicken and turkey), fish (especially fatty fish rich in omega-3s like salmon), and plant-based proteins (tofu, legumes).

Healthy Fats:

1. Purpose: Supports overall health and may help reduce inflammation.
2. Examples: Olive oil, avocados, and nuts in moderation.

Probiotic-Rich Foods:

1. Purpose: Promotes a healthy gut microbiome and supports digestive health.

2. Examples: Yogurt (choose plain, low-fat varieties without added sugars), kefir, and fermented foods like sauerkraut and kimchi.

Low-Lactose Dairy:

1. Purpose: Provides calcium and essential nutrients with reduced risk of digestive discomfort.
2. Examples: Lactose-free milk, yogurt, and aged cheeses.

Soft, Cooked Fruits and Vegetables:

1. Purpose: Easier to digest compared to raw counterparts, reducing strain on the digestive system.
2. Examples: Cooked apples, carrots, and squash without skins.

Herbal Teas and Water:

1. Purpose: Hydration is crucial for softening stool and promoting regular bowel movements.
2. Examples: Water, herbal teas (like chamomile or peppermint).

Whole Grains and Fiber Supplements:

1. Purpose: Ensures adequate fiber intake, supporting digestive health.
2. Examples: Whole grain bread and cereals, and fiber supplements (under healthcare provider guidance).

Balanced Meals with Regularity:

1. Purpose: Maintains stable digestion and prevents overeating that can stress the digestive system.
2. Examples: Balanced meals consisting of lean protein, high-fiber carbohydrates, and healthy fats, consumed at regular intervals.

Hydration and Fluid Intake:

1. Purpose: Essential for softening stool and preventing constipation.
2. Examples: Aim for at least eight glasses of water daily, adjusting based on individual needs and activity levels.

Chapter 2: Breakfast Boosters

Soothing Oatmeal Variations

Oatmeal is a versatile and soothing option for those managing diverticulitis, offering soluble fiber that aids digestion and helps regulate bowel movements. Variations can include:

1. Classic Oatmeal: Cook rolled oats with water or lactose-free milk until creamy. Top with bananas, berries, or a drizzle of honey.

2. Applesauce Oatmeal: Stir unsweetened applesauce into cooked oatmeal for added fiber and natural sweetness. Sprinkle with cinnamon for flavor.

3. Pumpkin Pie Oatmeal: Mix canned pumpkin puree with cooked oats, add a dash of pumpkin pie spice, and sweeten with a touch of maple syrup.

4. Nut Butter Oatmeal: Swirl in a spoonful of almond or peanut butter into warm oatmeal for extra protein and healthy fats.

Gentle Smoothie Recipes

Smoothies are easy to digest and can be packed with nutrients beneficial for diverticulitis. Try these gentle recipes:

1. Berry Banana Smoothie: Blend spinach, frozen berries, banana, and lactose-free yogurt for a fiber-rich and creamy treat.

2. Pineapple Ginger Smoothie: Combine fresh pineapple chunks, grated ginger, spinach, and coconut water for a refreshing anti-inflammatory boost.

3. Green Goddess Smoothie: Blend kale, cucumber, avocado, and lemon juice with almond milk for a smooth, nutrient-dense drink.

4. Protein Power Smoothie: Mix silken tofu, spinach, mango, and a scoop of protein powder with almond milk for a satisfying post-workout option.

Easy-to-Digest Egg Dishes

Eggs are a good source of protein and can be gentle on the digestive system when prepared thoughtfully:

1. Scrambled Eggs: Cook eggs gently with a splash of lactose-free milk and top with fresh herbs like chives or parsley.

2. Soft-Boiled Eggs: Serve eggs boiled just until the whites are set but the yolks remain runny, paired with whole grain toast.

3. Egg Salad: Mash hard-boiled eggs with a dollop of Greek yogurt, mustard, and dill for a creamy, protein-packed spread.

4. Vegetable Frittata: Bake eggs with sautéed spinach, bell peppers, and zucchini for a nutrient-rich meal that's soft and easy to chew.

Soft Muffins and Bread Options

Opt for softer varieties of bread and muffins, which are easier to digest and less likely to irritate the digestive tract:

1. Banana Bread Muffins: Use ripe bananas to sweeten whole grain muffins, incorporating oats for added fiber.

2. Zucchini Bread: Grate zucchini into a batter of whole wheat flour, eggs, and cinnamon for a moist and nutritious loaf.

3. Whole Grain Rolls: Choose soft, whole grain rolls or buns for sandwiches, lightly toasted for added texture.

4. Gluten-Free Options: Explore gluten-free muffin and bread recipes using alternatives like almond flour or oat flour for a softer texture.

Chapter 3: Lunch and Light Bites

Hearty Soups and Broths

Soups and broths are comforting and can be packed with nutrients while being gentle on the digestive system:

1. Chicken and Vegetable Soup: Simmer chicken breast with carrots, celery, and spinach in a low-sodium broth for a nourishing meal.

2. Bone Broth: Slow-cooked bone broth is rich in collagen and soothing for the gut. Add vegetables and herbs for flavor.

3. Lentil Soup: Cook lentils with carrots, tomatoes, and spices in vegetable broth for a fiber-rich and satisfying option.

4. Miso Soup: Combine miso paste with tofu, seaweed, and green onions in hot water for a probiotic-rich Japanese-inspired broth.

Light and Refreshing Salads

Salads provide hydration, fiber, and essential nutrients in a light and digestible form:

1. Greek Salad: Toss cucumber, tomatoes, olives, and feta cheese with a lemon-olive oil dressing for a refreshing option.

2. Quinoa Salad: Mix cooked quinoa with bell peppers, cucumber, and fresh herbs, dressed with a light vinaigrette.

3. Spinach and Strawberry Salad: Combine fresh spinach leaves with sliced strawberries, almonds, and a balsamic dressing.

4. Chickpea Salad: Combine chickpeas with diced cucumber, red onion, and parsley, dressed with lemon juice and olive oil.

Easy-to-Digest Sandwiches and Wraps

Sandwiches and wraps can be made with softer bread and fillings that are gentle on the digestive system:

1. Turkey and Avocado Wrap: Spread mashed avocado on a whole grain wrap, add sliced turkey breast, spinach, and a sprinkle of lemon juice.

2. Egg Salad Sandwich: Mash hard-boiled eggs with Greek yogurt, mustard, and dill, serve on whole grain bread.

3. Hummus and Vegetable Wrap: Spread hummus on a whole grain wrap, add shredded carrots, cucumber, and baby spinach.

4. Tuna Salad Sandwich: Mix canned tuna with Greek yogurt, diced celery, and lemon juice, serve on whole wheat bread.

Gentle Grain Bowls

Grain bowls provide a balanced meal with whole grains, vegetables, and lean proteins in an easy-to-digest format:

1. Brown Rice Bowl: Serve cooked brown rice with steamed broccoli, grilled chicken breast, and a drizzle of tahini sauce.

2. Quinoa and Roasted Vegetable Bowl: Combine quinoa with roasted sweet potatoes, bell peppers, and chickpeas, topped with a light lemon-herb dressing.

3. Sushi Bowl: Mix sushi rice with diced cucumber, avocado, and raw salmon or tofu, drizzle with soy sauce and sesame seeds.

4. Warm Farro Bowl: Cook farro and toss with sautéed kale, roasted butternut squash, and crumbled feta cheese.

Chapter 4: Nourishing Dinners

Flavorful Chicken Dishes

Chicken is a lean protein option that can be prepared in various ways while being gentle on the digestive system:

1. Grilled Chicken Breast: Marinate chicken breast in herbs, lemon juice, and olive oil, then grill until tender and juicy.

2. Chicken Stir-Fry: Sauté chicken strips with bell peppers, broccoli, and snap peas in a light soy sauce or teriyaki sauce.

3. Baked Chicken Thighs: Season chicken thighs with garlic, paprika, and thyme, then bake until golden brown and cooked through.

4. Chicken and Vegetable Skewers: Thread chicken cubes with cherry tomatoes, zucchini, and mushrooms, then grill or bake for a flavorful meal.

Tender Beef and Pork Recipes

Selecting lean cuts and tender preparations can make beef and pork suitable for a diverticulitis-friendly diet:

1. Beef Tenderloin Medallions: Sear beef tenderloin medallions with a simple salt and pepper rub, served with steamed vegetables.

2. Pork Tenderloin with Apples: Roast pork tenderloin with sliced apples, onions, and a touch of cinnamon for a sweet and savory dish.

3. Ground Turkey or Chicken Meatballs: Mix ground poultry with oats, egg, and seasonings, bake until cooked through, and serve with marinara sauce.

4. Slow-Cooked Beef Stew: Use lean beef stew meat with carrots, potatoes, and herbs, cooked in a low-sodium beef broth until tender.

Fish and Seafood for Sensitive Stomachs

Fish and seafood are rich in omega-3 fatty acids and can be easily digestible options:

1. Baked Salmon Fillets: Season salmon with dill, lemon juice, and olive oil, then bake until flaky and serve with steamed vegetables.

2. Grilled Shrimp Skewers: Marinate shrimp in garlic, lime juice, and cilantro, then grill until opaque and serve with a side of quinoa.

3. Poached Cod: Simmer cod fillets in a broth with herbs and vegetables until tender, then serve with a squeeze of fresh lemon.

4. Tuna Salad: Mix canned tuna with Greek yogurt, celery, and lemon juice, serve on a bed of mixed greens or whole grain crackers.

Vegetarian and Vegan Options

Plant-based options provide fiber and nutrients without the added strain on the digestive system:

1. Quinoa Stuffed Bell Peppers: Fill bell peppers with quinoa, black beans, corn, and salsa, then bake until peppers are tender.

2. Vegetable Stir-Fry: Sauté tofu or tempeh with broccoli, bell peppers, and snow peas in a light soy sauce or ginger sauce.

3. Lentil Soup: Cook lentils with carrots, celery, and tomatoes in vegetable broth for a hearty and fiber-rich soup.

4. Chickpea Curry: Simmer chickpeas with coconut milk, tomatoes, and curry spices, serve over brown rice or quinoa.

Chapter 5: Side Dishes and Add-ons

Comforting Rice and Pasta Dishes

Rice and pasta can be comforting staples in a diverticulitis-friendly diet when prepared with easy-to-digest ingredients and cooked to tender perfection:

1. Brown Rice Pilaf: Brown rice, known for its fiber content, can be transformed into a soothing pilaf by cooking it with vegetable broth and adding finely chopped, well-cooked vegetables like carrots and bell peppers. The fiber aids in digestion and supports gut health.

2. Chicken and Rice Casserole: Combine cooked chicken breast with brown rice, a light chicken broth, and tender vegetables such as peas and carrots. Bake until the flavors meld together for a comforting and nutritious meal.

3. Pasta Primavera: Opt for whole wheat or gluten-free pasta and cook until soft. Toss with lightly steamed vegetables like zucchini, bell peppers, and spinach, and add a splash of olive oil and a sprinkle of Parmesan cheese for added flavor without heavy sauces.

4. Creamy Mushroom Risotto: Arborio rice cooked slowly in a low-sodium vegetable broth with finely chopped mushrooms and a touch of lactose-free milk creates a creamy and digestible dish that's gentle on the stomach.

Soft Vegetable Sides

Incorporating soft vegetable sides ensures adequate fiber intake while being gentle on the digestive system:

1. Mashed Sweet Potatoes: Steam or bake sweet potatoes until tender, then mash with a bit of olive oil or butter. Sweet potatoes are rich in vitamins and fiber, promoting digestive health.

2. Steamed Carrots: Carrots can be steamed until soft and seasoned lightly with herbs like dill or parsley. Their natural sweetness makes them a delightful and digestible side.

3. Butternut Squash Puree: Roast butternut squash until soft, then puree with a splash of vegetable broth. This smooth and nutritious side is rich in vitamins and easy on the digestive tract.

4. Sautéed Spinach: Lightly sauté fresh spinach with garlic and a touch of olive oil until wilted. Spinach provides essential nutrients and is gentle when cooked thoroughly.

Simple and Digestible Legumes

Legumes can be included in a diverticulitis diet if prepared in a way that is easy to digest:

1. Lentil Soup: Cook lentils with carrots, celery, and low-sodium vegetable broth until soft. Pureeing the soup can make it even easier to digest while retaining all the nutritional benefits.

2. Hummus: Made from blended chickpeas, olive oil, lemon juice, and tahini, hummus is a creamy and protein-rich dip that pairs well with soft vegetables or whole grain crackers.

3. Split Pea Puree: Cook split peas until very tender and blend with a bit of vegetable broth to create a smooth and nourishing puree.

4. Black Bean Mash: Cook black beans until soft, then mash with garlic, cumin, and a splash of lime juice for a fiber-rich side dish.

Gut-Friendly Sauces and Dressings

Creating light and gut-friendly sauces and dressings can add flavor without causing irritation:

1. Olive Oil and Lemon Dressing: Mix extra virgin olive oil with fresh lemon juice, a pinch of salt, and pepper for a simple and refreshing salad dressing.

2. Yogurt Dill Sauce: Combine lactose-free Greek yogurt with fresh dill, lemon juice, and a pinch of garlic powder for a tangy and digestive-friendly sauce that pairs well with chicken or fish.

3. Avocado Lime Sauce: Blend ripe avocado with lime juice, cilantro, and a bit of water until smooth. This creamy sauce is perfect for drizzling over grilled vegetables or grain bowls.

4. Basil Pesto: Make a light pesto with fresh basil, spinach, a small amount of pine nuts, garlic, and olive oil. Use sparingly to add flavor to pasta or as a spread.

Chapter 6: Snacks and Small Plates

Easy-to-Digest Snack Ideas

Managing diverticulitis involves choosing snacks that are easy on the digestive system while providing essential nutrients. Some easy-to-digest options include:

1. Yogurt with Berries: Opt for lactose-free Greek yogurt topped with soft, ripe berries. This combination offers probiotics and fiber without being too harsh on the stomach.

2. Banana and Almond Butter: A ripe banana paired with a tablespoon of almond butter provides a mix of potassium and healthy fats, perfect for a gentle and satisfying snack.

3. Smoothies: Blend lactose-free milk or almond milk with soft fruits like bananas, mangoes, and spinach. Add a scoop of protein powder for a nutritious, drinkable snack.

Soft and Gentle Finger Foods

Soft finger foods are ideal for those needing to minimize digestive strain while enjoying satisfying snacks:

1. Avocado Toast: Mash avocado onto a slice of soft whole grain bread. Season with a pinch of salt and lemon juice for a nutritious and digestible snack.

2. Steamed Edamame: Lightly steamed edamame pods sprinkled with a bit of sea salt offer a soft, protein-rich snack that's easy on the digestive tract.

3. Soft Cheese and Crackers: Pair soft cheeses like ricotta or cottage cheese with whole grain crackers. This combination provides protein and fiber in an easily digestible form.

Healthy and Light Appetizers

Light appetizers can be both nutritious and easy to digest, perfect for small meals or snacks:

1. Cucumber Bites: Slice cucumbers and top with a dollop of Greek yogurt and a sprinkle of dill. These bites are hydrating, light, and easy to digest.

2. Zucchini Fritters: Grate zucchini and mix with egg and a small amount of flour, then lightly pan-fry until golden. These fritters are soft and gentle on the stomach.

3. Soft Boiled Eggs: Serve soft-boiled eggs with a sprinkle of salt and pepper. Eggs provide high-quality protein in a form that's easy to digest.

On-the-Go Snack Options

For those with busy lifestyles, having convenient and digestible snacks on hand is essential:

1. Fruit Cups: Pack single-serving fruit cups with soft fruits like peaches, pears, or applesauce. Ensure they are free from added sugars for a healthy snack.

2. Whole Grain Muffins: Bake whole grain muffins with ingredients like bananas or zucchini to ensure they are moist and easy to chew. These are perfect for a quick, portable snack.

3. Nut Butter Packets: Single-serving packets of almond or peanut butter can be paired with a banana or whole grain crackers for a convenient, protein-rich snack on the go.

Chapter 7: Desserts and Sweet Treats

Gentle Baked Goods

Baked goods can be part of a diverticulitis-friendly diet when made with the right ingredients and prepared to be easy on the digestive system:

1. Oatmeal Banana Muffins: Made with ripe bananas, oats, and a touch of honey, these muffins are moist, fiber-rich, and gentle on the stomach. Use whole grain or gluten-free flour to keep them light and easy to digest.

2. Applesauce Bread: Replace oil with unsweetened applesauce in a simple bread recipe. This swap not only reduces fat but also keeps the bread moist and soft, making it easier to chew and digest.

3. Zucchini Bread: Incorporate grated zucchini into a whole wheat or almond flour batter for a moist, fiber-rich treat. The zucchini adds moisture and nutrients without causing digestive discomfort.

Light and Refreshing Desserts

Desserts can be light, refreshing, and suitable for a sensitive digestive system:

1. Fruit Sorbet: Blend frozen berries or mango with a splash of water or coconut milk until smooth. This dairy-free dessert is cooling, hydrating, and gentle on the digestive tract.
2. Lemon Yogurt Parfait: Layer lactose-free Greek yogurt with lemon zest, a drizzle of honey, and soft, ripe berries. This parfait offers probiotics and a refreshing, tangy flavor.
3. Chia Seed Pudding: Mix chia seeds with almond milk and a touch of vanilla extract. Let it sit overnight to thicken, creating a creamy, fiber-rich pudding that is easy to digest.

Easy-to-Digest Fruit-Based Treats

Fruit-based treats can provide natural sweetness and essential nutrients while being gentle on the digestive system:

1. Baked Apples: Core and slice apples, sprinkle with cinnamon, and bake until soft. This warm treat is naturally sweet and easy to chew, perfect for a soothing dessert.

2. Peach Compote: Cook sliced peaches with a splash of water and a bit of honey until they break down into a soft compote. Serve over yogurt or oatmeal for added flavor and fiber.

3. Berry Smoothie Bowl: Blend soft fruits like bananas and berries with almond milk until smooth. Top with a few soft granola clusters or chia seeds for texture.

Indulgent Yet Safe Sweet Options

Even with dietary restrictions, it's possible to enjoy indulgent treats that are safe for diverticulitis:

1. Dark Chocolate Avocado Mousse: Blend ripe avocado with a bit of dark cocoa powder and honey until smooth. This mousse is rich, creamy, and full of healthy fats that are gentle on the stomach.

2. Coconut Macaroons: Make macaroons using shredded coconut, egg whites, and a touch of honey. These cookies are light, naturally sweet, and easy to digest.

3. Rice Pudding: Cook rice with almond milk, a bit of vanilla extract, and a sprinkle of cinnamon. This creamy pudding is both comforting and gentle on the digestive system.

Chapter 8: Drinks and Beverages

Hydrating Herbal Teas

Hydration is crucial for managing diverticulitis, and herbal teas provide a soothing, caffeine-free option:

1. Chamomile Tea: Known for its anti-inflammatory properties, chamomile tea can help calm the digestive system and reduce symptoms of discomfort. Drink it warm or chilled for a relaxing, hydrating experience.

2. Ginger Tea: Fresh ginger slices steeped in hot water create a tea that aids digestion and reduces nausea. Its natural anti-inflammatory effects can soothe the gut.

3. Peppermint Tea: Peppermint tea helps relax the muscles of the gastrointestinal tract, easing symptoms like bloating and gas. It's best enjoyed after meals to aid digestion.

Smooth and Gentle Smoothies

Smoothies can be nutrient-dense and easy to digest, making them ideal for a diverticulitis diet:

1. Banana and Oat Smoothie: Blend ripe bananas with cooked oats and a splash of almond milk. This smoothie is rich in fiber and potassium, supporting gut health and overall hydration.

2. Berry Spinach Smoothie: Combine spinach, blueberries, and lactose-free yogurt in a blender. The spinach provides essential vitamins, while the blueberries add antioxidants, creating a smooth and gentle drink.

3. Mango Coconut Smoothie: Blend fresh mango with coconut milk for a creamy, hydrating smoothie rich in vitamins A and C, essential for immune support and digestive health.

Nourishing Broths and Soups

Broths and soups offer hydration and essential nutrients while being gentle on the digestive system:

1. Bone Broth: Rich in collagen and minerals, bone broth supports gut health and provides a soothing, warm beverage that's easy to digest.

2. Vegetable Broth: Simmer carrots, celery, and zucchini in water with herbs like parsley and thyme. Strain the vegetables to create a clear, nutrient-rich broth that's gentle on the stomach.

3. Chicken Soup: Classic chicken soup made with tender chicken pieces, carrots, and noodles in a light broth is both nourishing and easy to digest, making it a comforting choice for those with diverticulitis.

Diverticulitis-Friendly Beverages

Staying hydrated with the right beverages is essential for managing diverticulitis:

1. Coconut Water: Naturally hydrating and rich in electrolytes, coconut water is a gentle and refreshing option for maintaining hydration levels without added sugars or artificial ingredients.

2. Aloe Vera Juice: Known for its soothing properties, aloe vera juice can help reduce inflammation in the digestive

tract. Ensure it is free from added sugars and additives for the best benefits.

3. Decaffeinated Green Tea: Green tea is rich in antioxidants, and choosing a decaffeinated version can help avoid irritation while still providing hydration and health benefits.

Chapter 9: Meal Plans and Shopping Lists

7-Day Meal Plan for Beginners

A 7-day meal plan tailored for beginners can simplify the transition to a diverticulitis-friendly diet, providing structure and ease:

1. Day 1: Start with oatmeal and bananas for breakfast, a chicken and vegetable soup for lunch, and baked salmon with steamed broccoli for dinner.

2. Day 2: Begin with a smoothie made of spinach, bananas, and almond milk. For lunch, have a turkey and avocado wrap. Dinner can be a lentil soup with carrots and celery.

3. Day 3: Greek yogurt with berries for breakfast, a quinoa salad with cucumbers and tomatoes for lunch, and grilled chicken with sweet potato for dinner.

4. Day 4: Enjoy a mango smoothie for breakfast, a bowl of vegetable broth with soft vegetables for lunch, and baked cod with zucchini for dinner.

5. Day 5: Soft-boiled eggs and whole-grain toast for breakfast, a mixed greens salad with light dressing for lunch, and turkey meatballs with brown rice for dinner.

6. Day 6: A banana and almond butter toast for breakfast, a vegetable stir-fry for lunch, and chicken breast with mashed potatoes for dinner.

7. Day 7: Oatmeal with honey for breakfast, a lentil and vegetable stew for lunch, and grilled tilapia with quinoa for dinner.

Customizable Weekly Meal Plans

Customizable weekly meal plans allow flexibility and personalization based on individual dietary needs and preferences:

1. Choose Proteins: Rotate between chicken, turkey, fish, and plant-based proteins like lentils and tofu.

2. Incorporate Vegetables: Select a variety of easily digestible vegetables such as carrots, zucchini, and spinach.

3. Mix Grains: Include different grains like quinoa, brown rice, and whole grain pasta.

4. Plan Snacks: Incorporate easy-to-digest snacks like yogurt, smoothies, and soft fruits.

Essential Shopping Lists

Creating an essential shopping list ensures you have all necessary ingredients for a diverticulitis-friendly diet:

1. Proteins: Chicken breasts, turkey, fish, tofu, eggs.

Vegetables: Carrots, zucchini, spinach, sweet potatoes, avocados.

2. Fruits: Bananas, berries, apples, mangoes.

Grains and Legumes: Oatmeal, quinoa, brown rice, lentils.

3. Dairy and Alternatives: Greek yogurt, almond milk, lactose-free cheese.

4. Miscellaneous: Olive oil, herbs, spices, low-sodium broths.

Tips for Meal Prep and Storage

Effective meal prep and storage can make following a diverticulitis diet more manageable and less time-consuming:

1. Batch Cooking: Prepare large batches of soups, stews, and grains that can be portioned out for the week.

2. Use Containers: Invest in quality containers for storing prepped meals and snacks. Label them with dates to ensure freshness.

3. Freeze Portions: Freeze individual portions of cooked proteins and soups for quick, easy meals on busy days.

4. Plan Ahead: Dedicate a day each week to plan meals, grocery shop, and prep ingredients to streamline your week.

Chapter 10: Diverticulitis Diet Recipes

Steamed Vegetable and Chicken Stir-Fry

Ingredients

• 1 Boneless, skinless chicken breast, cut into bite sized pieces

• 2 Tablespoons Olive Oil

• 2 Cloves of minced garlic

• 1 Diced onion

• 1 Diced bell pepper

• 2 Cups Diced mixed vegetables (broccoli, carrots, and zucchini)

• 1/4 Teaspoon salt

• 1/4 Teaspoon Black pepper

• 2 Tablespoons low-sodium soy sauce

• 2 Tablespoons cornstarch

• 2 Tablespoons water

• 2 Tablespoons chopped fresh parsley (optional)

Instructions

1. In a small bowl, whisk together the soy sauce, cornstarch, and water to make a stir-fry sauce.

2. In a large skillet, heat the olive oil over medium-high heat. Add the garlic, onion, bell pepper, mixed vegetables, salt, and black pepper. Stir-fry for 3-4 minutes, or until the vegetables are tender.

3. Push the vegetables to one side of the skillet and add the chicken. Stir-fry for 2-3 minutes, or until the chicken is cooked through.

4. Pour the stir-fry sauce over the chicken and vegetables and toss to coat. Cook for 1-2 minutes more, or until the sauce thickens.

5. Serve the stir-fry over steamed brown rice, and garnish with fresh parsley if desired.

Ziti with Zesty Chicken

Ingredients
- 1 Pound whole wheat ziti pasta or bowtie pasta
- 2 Teaspoons olive oil

- 1 onion, chopped

- 1 Tablespoon Dijon mustard

- 2 Tablespoons whole wheat flour

- 2 Cups chicken broth

- 1/4 Cup lemon juice

- 12 Ounces frozen peas, thawed

- 1/4 Cup fresh Italian parsley, chopped

- 12 Ounces cooked chicken, chopped

Instructions

1. Bring a large pot of salted water to a boil. Add pasta and cook according to package instructions until al dente. Drain.

2. While pasta is cooking, in a large non-stick pan, heat olive oil over medium heat. Add the onion and cook for 3 minutes. Stir in the Dijon mustard and flour. Gradually whisk in the chicken broth, stirring constantly to avoid clumps.

3. Bring the broth to a boil and stir in the lemon juice, peas and parsley. Add cooked pasta and cooked chicken to sauce and serve.

Beef and Penne Pasta Toss

• Cuisine: Pasta

• Course: Main Dishes

• Serves: 4

Ingredients

• 1 Pound whole wheat penne pasta

• 1 Pound ground beef, lean

• 2 Tablespoons olive oil

• 1 small onion, chopped

• 3 garlic cloves, minced

• 15 Ounces can tomatoes, seeded, diced

• 2 Cups medium zucchini, seeded, chopped

• 8 Ounces fresh spinach, chopped

• 1 Cup Parmesan cheese, grated

Instructions

1. Bring a large pot of salted water to a boil. Cook penne pasta al dente according to package directions.

2. In a large non-stick pan, brown ground beef over medium-high heat for 6 to 8 minutes, breaking up any large

pieces. Remove beef and set aside on paper towels to drain excess fat.

3. In the same pan, heat olive oil over medium-high heat. Cook onions and garlic for about 5 minutes or until soft. Add tomatoes and zucchini and continue cooking 5 minutes more. Add spinach and cook until it just wilts, 2-3 minutes.

4. Return beef to skillet and stir in 1/2 cup cheese; heat through Transfer pasta to a large serving bowl and spoon meat mixture on top.

5. Toss until well combined and sprinkle with remaining cheese.

Delicious Sweet Potatoes

• Course Holiday Recipes
• Serves: 6-8

Ingredients

• 4 Pounds sweet potatoes, peeled and cut into large bite size pieces
• 2 Cups orange juice

- 1/2 Cup honey

- 1 Teaspoon cinnamon

- 1 Teaspoon nutmeg

- 2 Tablespoons vanilla extract

- 2 Teaspoons lemon zest

- 2 Tablespoons flour

- 1/2 Cup brown sugar

Instructions

1. Preheat oven to 350 degrees. Boil sweet potatoes until slightly underdone. Drain, cool and set aside. In a large bowl, whisk together orange juice, cinnamon, nutmeg, vanilla and zest. In another bowl, combine flour and both sugar together. Put cooled sweet potatoes in a deep baking dish, add dry ingredient mixture and stir to coat. Pour liquid over sweet potatoes and bake for 20 to 25 minutes.

White Bean Puree

- Course: Snacks

- Serves: 4

Ingredients

- 14 Ounces cannellini beans, drained and rinsed
- 2 garlic cloves
- 1/4 Cup fresh Italian parsley
- 1/2 lemon, juiced
- 1/4 Teaspoon oregano
- 1/2 Teaspoon salt
- 1/3 Cup olive oil

Instructions

1. Blend all ingredients in a food processor until almost smooth. Serve with crusty bread, whole wheat crackers, or fresh vegetables

Easy Turkey Chili

- Course Main Dishes
- Serves: 4-6

Ingredients

- 3 Tablespoons olive oil

- Garlic cloves, minced
- Onion, chopped
- 1 Pound ground turkey
- Bay leaf
- 1 Teaspoon ground cumin
- 1 Teaspoon dried oregano
- Tomato, seeded, chopped
- 14 Ounces can tomato sauce
- 1 Cup beef broth
- 1 Teaspoon salt
- 28 Ounces can red beans, drained and rinsed

Instructions

1. In a large pot, heat oil over medium heat and cook garlic and onions for a 5 minutes.

2. Increase heat to high and add turkey, bay leaf, cumin and oregano. Cook until turkey has browned, about 5-7 minutes.

3. Add tomato, tomato sauce, broth and salt. Bring pot to a boil and then lower heat to simmer. Cover and simmer for about 20 minutes.

4. Add beans and more water if needed, and continue to simmer for 25 more minutes. Serve.

Baked Lemon Garlic Salmon Recipe

• Total Time: 28 minutes
• Yield: Serves 6

INGREDIENTS
For Salmon:
• 2 lb salmon fillet
• Kosher salt
• Extra virgin olive oil (I used Early Harvest Greek extra virgin olive oil)
• ½ lemon, sliced into rounds
• Parsley for garnish
For Lemon-Garlic Sauce:
• Zest of 1 large lemon
• Juice of 2 lemons
• 3 tbsp extra virgin olive oil (I used Early Harvest Greek extra virgin olive oil)
• 5 garlic cloves, chopped

- 2 tsp dry oregano

- 1 tsp sweet paprika

- ½ tsp black pepper

INSTRUCTIONS

1. Heat oven to 375 degrees F.

2. Make the lemon-garlic sauce. In a small bowl or measuring cup, mix together the lemon juice, lemon zest, extra virgin olive oil, garlic, oregano, paprika and black pepper. Give the sauce a good whisk.

3. Prepare a sheet pan lined with a large piece of foil (should be large enough to fold over salmon). Brush top of the foil with extra virgin olive oil.

4. Now, pat salmon dry and season well on both sides with kosher salt. Place it on the foiled sheetpan. Top with lemon garlic sauce (make sure to spread the sauce evenly.)

5. Fold foil over the salmon (seam-side up). Bake for 15 to 20 minutes until salmon is almost completely cooked through at the thickest part (cooking time will vary based on the thickness of your fish. If your salmon is thinner, check several minutes early to ensure your salmon does not

overcook. If your piece is very thick, 1 ½ or more inches, it may take a bit longer.)

6. Carefully remove from oven and open foil to uncover the top of the salmon. Place under the broiler briefly, about 3 minutes or so. Watch closely as it broils to make sure it doesn't overcook and the garlic does not burn).

Easy Beef Stir Fry

• Course Main Dishes

• Serves: 2-3

Ingredients

• 1/4 Cup orange juice

• 1/4 Cup low-sodium soy sauce

• 2 Tablespoons rice vinegar

• 1/4 Cup water

• 2 Tablespoons canola oil

• 8 Ounces beef round tip steak, thinly sliced

• Garlic cloves, minced

• 6 Ounces peas, thawed from frozen

• Bunch broccoli florets

• 8 Ounces edamame, shelled

• 1 1/2 Teaspoon cornstarch, dissolved in 1/4 C warm water

Instructions

1. In a small bowl, combine orange juice, soy sauce, rice vinegar, and water until well combined. Set aside.

2. In a large non-stick pan, heat 1 tablespoon of canola oil over medium-high heat. Add the beef and cook, stirring, until just browned, about 2 minutes. Transfer the beef to a separate plate.

3. Heat another tablespoon of oil over medium heat and cook garlic about 1 minute, without burning it. Add peas, broccoli and edamame, and continue to cook for 3 minutes.

4. Add the soy sauce mixture and cook, stirring, until broccoli is cooked and crisp-tender, about 5 minutes.

5. Add the sliced beef back into pan and add dissolved cornstarch in water and stir to combine all ingredients.

6. Cook until mixture thickens slightly and beef is heated through. Serve immediately.

Low FODMAP French Oven Beef Stew

PREP TIME: 15 minutes

COOK TIME: 4 hours

TOTAL TIME: 4 hours hrs 15 minutes

COURSE: Main Dish

SERVINGS: 6 servings

INGREDIENTS

- 1 lb beef for stew
- 1 cup fennel bulb , diced
- 1 medium celery stalks
- 6 medium carrots
- 4 medium parsnips
- 4 medium potatoes
- 1/4 cup tapioca quick cooking
- 1 cup tomato juice
- 1 Tbsp sugar (optional)
- ½ tsp salt
- ½ tsp freshly ground pepper
- 1 tsp ground basil

INSTRUCTIONS

• Preheat oven to 300°F. Cut the beef into approximately 4 cm/1 ½ inch cubes.

• Wash all vegetables well. Scrub potato skin to remove all dirt. Medium dice celery stalks and fennel bulb. Chop carrots, parsnips and potatoes into medium sized pieces.

• Mix all ingredients EXCEPT potatoes in a large oven-safe dish with a lid. Cover and bake in oven for 3 hours.

• Mix in potatoes and bake for 1 hour longer. Enjoy.

NOTES

• Make sure to purchase tomato juice WITHOUT added onion or garlic

• If your tomato juice is sodium-free, option to increase amount of salt to 1 tsp

• Fennel bulb is low FODMAP at 1/2 cup per serving. Celery is low FODMAP at 1/4 medium stalk per serving. There is 1 medium celery stalk in the stew and therefore the max FODMAP serving size is 1/4 of the recipe; this means that you could eat up to 1/4 of the total amount of stew and still stay low FODMAP.

Chicken Florentine

• Course: Main Dishes

• Serves: 4

Ingredients

• 2 Tablespoons olive oil

• 2 zucchinis, seeded, thinly sliced

• 1/2 Cup green onion, sliced

• 2 chicken breast, cubed

• 1/2 Teaspoon salt

• 1/2 Teaspoon thyme, ground

• 3 Cups long grain rice, cooked

• 4 Cups fresh spinach, chopped

• 1/4 Cup Parmesan cheese, grated

Instructions

1. In a medium pan, heat olive oil over medium heat.

2. Add zucchini, onions, and chicken, stirring occasionally for 5 to 10 minutes, or until chicken is golden.

3. Add salt, thyme, rice and spinach. Cook and stir for another 6 - 8 minutes or until heated through and spinach wilts.

4. Remove from heat, transfer to a large serving bowl, and stir in cheese. Serve.

Clear Soup Recipe (Clear Vegetable Soup)

INGREDIENTS

- 1 large yellow onion (avoid red onion)
- 1 cup celery stalks (you can also add more) chopped
- 2 carrots diced or cubed (can add more)
- 10 french beans (lesser if also fine)
- ½ cabbage diced
- 1 to 2 stalks celery leaves or coriander leaves
- 1½ cup mushrooms sliced (or ½ cup mixed veggies or broccoli).
- 8 florets cauliflower (optional)

Optional

- 1 tsp garlic chopped
- 1 tsp ginger chopped
- 1 tbsp oil
- 1 stalk spring onion greens or scallions
- ½ tsp crushed pepper or ground pepper

INSTRUCTIONS

Preparation (make vegetable stock)

• Add all the veggies except mushrooms & spring onions to a large pot.

• Pour water just enough to immerse them. I used 2½ cups of water.

• Cover and simmer on a low flame until the veggies wilt off completely and turn flavorless.

• Place a strainer over a large pot and strain the veggies.

• If you intend to eat the veggies then skip this step. Mash the veggies well & leave in the strainer for 20 mins. You will get about half cup soup.

How to Make Clear Soup

• Heat the same pan with oil.

• Saute ginger and garlic for a minute.

• Then add the mushrooms and saute well until they begin to smell good.

• Pour the strained clear soup to this and simmer until the mushrooms are done to your liking.

• If desired add some salt to taste. You can also serve the veggies on the side if you desire.

To make Chicken Clear Soup

• Add 250 grams bone-in chicken along with veggies & 3 cups water to the pot.

• Cook until the chicken falls off the bone.

• Remove the chicken aside and then strain the clear soup.

• Shred the chicken and set aside.

• Heat oil and saute ginger garlic until aromatic.

• Saute the shredded chicken and pour the clear soup. You can also saute mushrooms first and then add chicken.

• Let the soup come to a boil to bring out the flavors of ginger and garlic.

• Add spring onion greens and season with salt.

Tofu Stir Fry

• Course: Main Dishes
• Serves: 4

Ingredients

• 14 Ounces firm tofu, drained, patted dry and cut into thick slices

• 1/4 Cup whole wheat flour

- 1 Tablespoon canola oil

- 1/2 Cup olive oil

- 2 Tablespoons balsamic vinegar

- 1 Tablespoon Dijon mustard

- 3 Tablespoons low sodium soy sauce

- 1/2 Cup onions, sliced

- 1/2 Cup carrots, sliced

- 1 Cup green beans, ends cut

- 1 Cup cabbage, chopped

- 1 Cup brown rice, cooked

Instructions

1. In a shallow bowl or plate, mix tofu with flour until evenly coated. In a non-stick pan, heat canola oil over medium-high heat. Add tofu and cook until lightly brown. Remove from pan and put aside.

2. Prepare dressing by whisking together olive oil, vinegar, mustard and soy sauce.

3. In same pan, combine 2 tablespoons of the dressing mixture with onions, carrots, green beans, soy beans and cabbage.

4. Stir fry for 10 minutes or until vegetables are tender. Add remaining dressing mixture and tofu. Mix. Cook for 2 minutes, stirring gently.

5. Serve over hot brown rice.

Greek White Bean and Feta Salad

- Course: Salads
- Serves: 6

Ingredients
- 2 Tablespoons plain yogurt
- 3 Tablespoons olive oil
- 2 Tablespoons fresh lemon juice
- 3/4 Teaspoons oregano
- 1 Tablespoon fresh mint, chopped
- 28 Ounces white cannellini beans, drained and rinsed
- 1/2 Cup red onion, chopped finely
- 3 medium tomatoes, seeded and chopped
- 1/4 Cup Greek olives, pitted
- 1/2 Cup feta cheese,crumbled
- 2 Cups fresh spinach leaves, torn

Instructions

1. In large bowl, combine yogurt, olive oil, lemon juice, oregano, and mint ; whisk well.

2. Add beans, onion, tomato, olives and feta cheese; toss lightly.

3. Refrigerate for at least one hour. Serve on a bed of spinach.

Summer Spaghetti

• Course Main Dishes

• Serves: 4

Ingredients

• 1 Pound whole wheat spaghetti

• 1/4 Cup olive oil

• Shallot, minced

• Garlic cloves, minced

• Medium zucchini, chopped

• Medium summer squash, chopped

• 1/4 Cup fresh basil, chopped

• 1/2 Teaspoon salt

* Medium lemon, juiced
* 2 Tablespoons butter, room temperature
* Freshly grated lemon peel

Instructions

1. Bring a large pot of salted water to boil. Add pasta and cook according to package directions until al dente.
2. In a large pan, heat oil over medium heat and cook the shallot and garlic stirring frequently.
3. Add the zucchini, squash, and basil. Continue to cook, stirring occasionally, until all vegetables are tender. Season with salt and lemon juice.
4. Immediately place the sautéed vegetables with all their juices in a large shallow pasta bowl.
5. Add the linguine and butter, toss to mix well and serve immediately. Top with freshly grated lemon peel.

Asparagus Soup

* Course Soups
* Serves: 4

Ingredients

- 1 Tablespoon olive oil

- 1 Cup shallots, finely chopped

- 3 garlic cloves, minced

- 2 Pounds asparagus, chopped into one inch pieces

- 6 Cups vegetable stock

- 1 Teaspoon salt

Instructions

1. Reserve asparagus tops for later use. In a large soup pot, heat olive oil over medium heat. Cook shallots and garlic until softened, about 3-5 minutes.

2. Add asparagus stalks, vegetable stock and salt and bring to a boil. Cover and reduce heat to low and simmer until asparagus softens.

3. Let soup cool and puree with a hand blender, until creamy. Add asparagus tops and cook on medium for 5 minutes, until tops are tender.

BEST CLEAR CHICKEN SOUP (BROTH RECIPE)

PREP TIME: 30 minutes

COOK TIME: 2 hours

TOTAL TIME: 2 hours 30 minutes

INGREDIENTS

• 2 chicken quarters around 1 kg (2.2 lb) of chicken; see notes for different cuts of chicken you can use

• 2 onions

• 1 celery stalk

• 2 celeriac (100 g or 3.5oz)

• 2 parsnips or parsely roots

• 5 carrots

• 1 kale leaf

• Bunch parsely

• 1 tbsp fine salt

• 5 l water 22 cups

INSTRUCTIONS

• Remove the chicken from the packaging; take a large stockpot, place the chicken in and add 5 litres/ 21 US cups of water.

• Bring to boil. When it starts boiling the dark grey impurities will start rising to the top and then you start removing it with a fine mesh food strainer (or spoon). This will last about 10-20 minutes depending on the chicken. Once the water seems mostly clear (no grey) you can add the vegetables.

• Add the vegetables and salt and bring to boil. Once boiling, reduce to the lowest heat, cover and simmer the soup for a minimum of 2 hours or however long you want. You can let it simmer for the whole day, it will just be tastier and the chicken will be so soft.

• Once the 2 hours pass, take a pot that is a similar size and drain the soup.

• The chicken should be falling off the bones. You can always heat up some homemade or store-bought noodles and add to the soup.

• Store in fridge for up to 3 days and in the freezer for up to 3 months.

NOTES

• If you don't have a fine mesh food strainer use a spoon and just add more water when you add the vegetables

• It can also be made with a whole chicken, bone-in chicken thighs or any part fo the chicken with bones.

• Instead of chicken you can use beef and the same vegetables

• The longer you cook the soup the more flavor it will have. A minimum is 2 hours but you can keep it going for 6 or more

• Cook with as many carrots as you want to eat

• To serve clear chicken soup to baby place it in a cup and let then drink it. To cool it quickly add an ice cube in and wait until it melts

Black Bean Quesadillas

• Course: Main Dishes
• Serves: 4

Ingredients

- 1 Tablespoon olive oil

- 1/2 small onion, chopped

- 1/2 Cup red bell pepper, seeded, chopped

- 1 clove, minced

- 28 Ounces black beans, rinsed, drained, lightly mashed

- 1/2 Teaspoon cumin

- 3 Tablespoons cilantro, chopped

- 1/4 Cup black olives, sliced

- 2 Cups fresh spinach, chopped

- 3/4 Cups Monterey Jack cheese, shredded

- 8 whole wheat tortillas

Instructions

1. Preheat oven to 350 degrees.

2. In a medium pan, heat olive oil over medium heat. Cook onions and red peppers until soft, about 5 minutes. Add garlic and continue to cook another 2 minutes, add mashed beans, cilantro and olives, and cumin and cook another 5 minutes to combine all ingredients.

3. Spread mixture evenly onto 4 tortillas. Sprinkle with spinach and cheese.

4. Top with remaining tortillas. Bake tortillas on ungreased cookie sheet for 12 minutes. Cut into wedges and serve.

Low FODMAP Pad Thai with Shrimp

- Prep Time: 15 minutes
- Cook Time: 15 minutes
- Category: Main Dish
- Method: Skillet, Stovetop

Ingredients

- 8 ounces uncooked rice noodles, such as Thai Kitchen Brown Rice Noodles
- ¼ cup granulated sugar
- 2 tablespoons plain rice vinegar
- 2 tablespoons reduced-sodium soy sauce (or tamari for gluten-free)
- 1 tablespoon fish sauce
- 2 teaspoons ground paprika
- 2 tablespoons+1 teaspoon garlic-infused olive oil, divided
- 1 medium (225 grams) green bell pepper, thinly sliced
- 1.5 cups shredded green cabbage

• 1 pound (454 grams) uncooked medium or large shrimp, peeled and deveined

• ½ cup sliced green onion tops (green parts only)

• 1 large egg, whisked – optional

• Chopped fresh cilantro leaves – optional garnish

INSTRUCTIONS

1. Check the rice noodle package instructions. If directed, start boiling the cooking water.

2. In a small bowl, whisk together sugar, rice vinegar, soy sauce (or tamari), fish sauce, and paprika.

3. Heat 2 tablespoons garlic-infused oil in a large skillet over medium heat. Once the oil is hot, add the bell pepper slices and cabbage. Cook for 3 to 5 minutes or until the veggies start to soften.

4. While the peppers cook, prepare the rice noodles according to the package instructions. Drain.

5. Once the peppers start to soften, add the shrimp to the skillet. Cook for 2 to 4 minutes or until the shrimp start to turn opaque pink and are almost cooked through. Add the sauce and cook for about 1 minute or until the shrimp are cooked and the sugar has dissolved. Reduce the heat to low.

6. Stir in the noodles and green onion tops. Cook until everything is hot. Then, remove from the heat.

7. Optional: Heat the remaining 1 teaspoon of garlic-infused oil over medium-high heat in a small nonstick skillet. Once hot, add the egg and cook, scrambling with a silicone spatula, until done. Stir into the noodle mixture.

8. Serve warm, topped with optional cilantro leaves.

NOTES

1. Low FODMAP Serving: One serving of this recipe (¼ recipe/about 1.5 cups/225 grams) uses low FODMAP amounts of ingredients at the date of publication. Individual tolerance may vary, and low FODMAP servings may change. For more information on specific ingredients, please refer to the Monash FODMAP App or check out the "FODMAP Notes" section (above the recipe).

2. Fish sauce: Add more to taste, up to 2 tablespoons per serving.

Asian Chicken Salad

• Course Salads

• Serves: 1

Ingredients

• 1 Cup romaine lettuce, chopped

• 1 carrot, shredded

• 1 celery, sliced thinly

• 1/4 Cup red bell pepper, seeded, sliced thinly

• 1/2 Cup chicken breast, cut into strips

• 1/4 Cup mangoes

• 2 Tablespoons lime and ginger dressing, store bought

Instructions

1. In a medium bowl, toss together all ingredients until combined.

2. Serve alone or with whole wheat bread slices.

Quinoa Tabbouleh (Low FODMAP)

Ingredients

- 500 ml (2 cups) water
- 250 ml (1 cup) quinoa
- 2 Roma tomatoes
- 1 English cucumber
- 1 bunch curly parsley
- 3 green onions, green part only
- 30 ml (2 tbsp) olive oil
- The juice of one lemon
- Pepper and salt, to taste

Preparation

1. Place water and quinoa with a pinch of salt in a saucepan. Bring to a boil and reduce to a simmer for 10 to 15 minutes or until the liquid is completely absorbed.

2. Chill quinoa in refrigerator (or freeze for a quicker option).

3. Dice tomatoes and cucumbers. Finely chop parsley and green onion.

4. Mix quinoa with vegetables, herbs, oil and lemon juice. Season with salt and pepper to taste.

5. Serve the salad with grilled meat or fish.

Baked Salmon with Vegetable Quinoa

• Course Main Dishes

Ingredients

• 4 Salmon fillets

• 1/4 Teaspoon Salt

• 1/4 Teaspoon Black pepper

• 1 Tablespoon Olive oil

• 1 Cup Quinoa

• 2 Cups Vegetable broth

• 1 Diced onion

• 2 Cloves of minced garlic

• 1 Diced bell pepper

• 1 Diced zucchini

• 1/4 Cup Chopped fresh parsley

• 2 Teaspoons Lemon juice

Instructions

1. Preheat the oven to 375°F (190°C)

2. Season the salmon fillets with salt and pepper.

3. Heat the olive oil in a skillet over medium heat. Add the salmon fillets and cook for 2-3 minutes per side, or until golden brown.

4. Transfer the salmon to a baking dish and bake in the preheated oven for 8-10 minutes, or until cooked through.Meanwhile, rinse the quinoa in a fine mesh strainer and drain.

5. In a saucepan, bring the vegetable broth to a boil. Add the quinoa and return to a boil. Reduce the heat to low, cover, and simmer for 18-20 minutes, or until the quinoa is cooked and the broth is absorbed.

6. In the same skillet, sauté the onion, garlic, bell pepper, and zucchini until they are tender. Stir in the cooked quinoa, parsley, and lemon juice.

7. Serve the baked salmon with the vegetable quinoa on the side.

Brown Rice Greek Salad

• Course Salads

• Serves: 2

Ingredients

- 1/2 Cup Brown rice, cooked
- 1/2 Cup white beans, canned, drained, rinsed
- 1/2 Cup fresh spinach
- 1/2 Cup tomatoes, no seeds
- 1/2 Cup English Cucumber, no seeds
- 1/4 Cup avocado, diced
- 1 Tablespoon red onion, chopped
- 2 Tablespoons Feta cheese, crumbled
- 2 Tablespoons extra virgin olive oil
- 1 Teaspoon red wine vinegar
- to taste salt and pepper
-

Instructions

1. In a medium bowl, combine brown rice, beans, spinach, tomatoes, cucumber, avocado, onion, and cheese until combined.

2. Drizzle oil and vinegar on top and season to taste with salt and pepper and toss together.

3. Can be served alone or with whole wheat pita bread.

Vegeterian Penne Pasta

- Cuisine Pastavegetarian
- Course Main Dishes
- Serves: 2

Ingredients

- 1/2 Pound whole wheat penne or bowtie pasta
- 1 Tablespoon salt
- 2 Tablespoons olive oil
- 8 Ounces white mushrooms, sliced
- 8 Ounces asparagus, chopped
- 8 Ounces red bell pepper, seeded and chopped
- 1/4 Cup Parmesan cheese, grated
- 1/4 Cup fresh basil, chopped

Instructions

1. Bring a large pot of salted water to boil. Add pasta and cook according to package directions until al dente. Drain.
2. While the pasta is cooking, in a medium non-stick pan, heat olive oil over medium heat. Add the mushrooms and cook for about five minutes to release all the water.

3. Add the asparagus and bell pepper and sauté for 3-4 minutes, until softened. Add cooked pasta to pan and add Parmesan cheese, stir until well combined.

4. Transfer to a serving bowl, garnish with fresh basil and serve.

Grilled Vegetable Quesadilla

• Course Main Dishes

Ingredients

• Zucchini, sliced in half, lengthwise

• Yello squash, sliced in half lengthwise

• Onion, sliced in fourths, lenghtwise

• Red pepper, seeded and quartered

• Portobello mushroom cap

• 1/2 Teaspoon Italian seasoning

• 1/4 Teaspoon salt

• Whole wheat tortillas

• 1/2 Cup Mozzarella cheese, shredded

Instructions

1. Grill vegetables over medium heat until all of the vegetables are cooked. Season with Italian seasoning and salt. Slice vegetables and toss together.

2. Heat a pan sprayed with non-stick cooking spray over medium heat and place one tortilla in the pan. Spread some of the vegetable mixture over the tortilla, sprinkle with cheese and top with the remaining tortilla. Turn tortilla over and heat the other side until cheese melts but do not brown the tortillas. Serve.

Slow cooker gut-healing chicken soup

• Prep: 45m

• Cook: 6h 55m

• Serves: 6

Ingredients

• 2 tbsp olive oil

• 1 leek, halved, thinly sliced

• 1 brown onion, finely chopped

• 2 carrots, peeled, cut into 2cm piece

• 2 celery sticks, sliced

- 3 garlic cloves, crushed

- 350g sweet potato, peeled, cut into 2cm pieces

- 2 (about 370g) parsnips, peeled, cut into 2cm pieces

- 2 zucchini, chopped

- 3/4 cup fresh continental parsley leaves, chopped

- 2 lemons, rind finely grated, juiced

- 60g baby spinach

- Crusty wholegrain bread, to serve (optional)

- Soup base

- 1.8kg whole organic or free-range chicken

- 1 brown onion, halved

- 1 carrot, halved

- 1 celery stick, halved

- 2 fresh bay leaves

- 4 fresh continental parsley sprigs

- 1 tbsp apple cider vinegar

- 1L (4 cups) Massel salt reduced chicken style liquid stock

Method

- To make soup base, place soup base, brown onion, carrot, celery, bay leaves, parsley, apple cider vinegar and stock in a 5.5L slow cooker. Pour in enough water to just cover. Set to Low. Cook, covered, for 3 hours

• Meanwhile, heat oil in a saucepan over medium-low heat. Cook leek, onion, carrot, celery and garlic for 10-12 minutes or until softened.

• Transfer leek mixture to slow cooker. Cook, covered, for 2 1 /2 hours. Add sweet potato and parsnip. Cover. Cook for a further 30 minutes or until chicken is very tender and falling off the bone.

• Transfer chicken to a bowl. Use tongs to remove and discard halved onion, carrot and celery, bay leaves and parsley sprigs. Shred chicken, discarding skin and bones. Return to the bowl. Cover to keep warm.

• Add the zucchini and chopped parsley to the slow cooker. Cook, covered, for 30-40 minutes or until vegetables are tender.

• Stir in chicken, lemon rind and juice. Season. Cover. Cook for 15 minutes. Remove from heat. Stir in spinach. Serve with bread, if using.

Holiday Stuffing

- Course: Holiday Recipes
- Serves: 4

Ingredients

- 1 loaf whole wheat bread, cubed
- 3/4 stick unsalted butter
- 3 large tart apples, unpeeled, chopped
- 1 onion, chopped
- 3 celery stalks, chopped
- 2 Cups chicken broth
- 1/2 Cup dried apricots
- 1/2 Cup prunes, chopped
- 1/2 Cup fresh Italian parsley
- 1/2 Tablespoon salt

Instructions

1. Preheat oven to 400 degrees. Lay cubed bread on a baking sheet in a single layer and bake, until toasted, about 10 minutes. Allow to cool. While bread is toasting, prepare fruit mixture. Heat butter in a large pan over medium- high heat. Add apples, onion, and celery and cook until softened,

about 8-10 minutes. Put mixture in a large bowl and combine with toasted bread, broth, apricots, prunes, parsley and salt. Transfer mixture to a 3-quart baking dish and cover with foil. Bake 20 minutes, remove foil and bake an additional 15 minutes

Spaghetti with Zucchini

• Cuisine: Pasta
• Course: Main Dishes
• Serves: 4

Ingredients
• 1 Pound whole wheat spaghetti
• 2 zucchini, grated, water squeezed out or spiraled
• 2 Tablespoons butter
• 1 Tablespoon olive oil
• Garlic cloves, minced
• 1/2 Cup Parmesan cheese, grated

Instructions

1. Bring a large pot of salted water to boil. Add pasta and cook according to package directions until al dente.

2. While pasta is cooking, in a large non-stick pan, heat butter and oil together. Add grated zucchini and cook for about 3 minutes. Add garlic and cook for one more minute, stirring constantly. Add 1/4 cup of grated parmesan cheese.

3. Place pasta in a large shallow pasta bowl and toss in zucchini mixture. Top with remaining parmesan cheese. Serve

Greek Yogurt Fettuccini Alfredo

1. Yield: Serves 8

2. Prep time: 10 minutes

3. Cook time: 15 minutes

4. Total time: 25 minutes

Ingredients

1. 1 pound fettuccini

2. 1½ cups whole-milk Greek yogurt

3. ½ cup freshly grated Parmesan, plus more for serving

4. 3 tablespoons minced garlic

5. ¼ cup chopped fresh parsley

6. 1 teaspoon pepper

Instructions

• Boil pasta in salted water per package instructions. Reserve 1 cup cooking liquid, then drain.

• Whisk together yogurt, ½ cup Parmesan, garlic, and parsley. Slowly whisk in cooking liquid a little bit at a time. Add pepper. Pour sauce over pasta and toss to combine.

• Top with more Parmesan to taste and serve immediately. Pasta should register 145 degrees Fahrenheit or higher using an instant-thermometer placed in the middle of the dish.

Mediterranean Salmon and Potato Salad

• Course: Salads

• Serves: 4

Ingredients

• 1 Pound red potatoes, unpeeled, cut into wedges

- 1/2 Cup olive oil

- 2 Tablespoons balsamic vinegar

- 1 Tablespoon rosemary, minced

- 2 Cups white cannellini beans, drained and rinsed

- 4 salmon fillets, 4 oz each

- 2 Tablespoons lemon juice

- 1/4 Teaspoon salt

- 8 large lettuce leaves, torn

- 2 Cups English cucumber, seedless, sliced

Instructions

1. In a medium saucepan, bring water to a boil and cook potatoes until tender, about 10 minutes. Drain and pour potatoes back into pan.

2. To make dressing, in a small bowl, whisk together 1/2 cup of olive oil, vinegar and rosemary. Combine potatoes and white beans with dressing. Set aside.

3. In a separate medium pan, heat the remaining 2 tbs of olive oil over medium-high heat. Add salmon fillets and sprinkle with lemon juice and salt. Cook about 5-7 minutes on each side or until fish flakes easily.

4. To serve, place lettuce and cucumber slices on a serving platter top with potato salad and fish fillets.

Sunrise Burrito Wrap

• Course: Breakfast

• Serves: 1 wrap

Ingredients

• 1 Tablespoon olive oil

• 2 Slices turkey

• 1/4 Cup green bell pepper, seeded, chopped

• 1/4 Cup black beans

• 2 eggs

• 2 Tablespoons milk

• 1/4 Teaspoon salt

• 2 Tablespoons Monterrey Jack cheese, grated

• 1 whole wheat tortilla

Instructions

1. In a small non-stick pan, heat olive oil on medium heat and cook turkey about 2 minutes until slightly crispy.

2. Add bell peppers and beans and continue to cook until warmed through.

3. In a small bowl beat together egg with milk and salt. Add beaten eggs and stir gently until eggs are almost cooked through.

4. Add grated cheese and lower heat to lowest setting. Cover and continue to cook until cheese has completely melted. Place mixture on wheat tortilla and roll into a burrito.

Beef and Vegetable Soup

• Course Soups

Ingredients
• 1/2 Pound stew beef, diced
• 1/2 bag frozen vegetable medley
• 1/4 Cup barley
• 32 Ounces beef broth
• 2 tomatoes, seeded and chopped
• 1 Teaspoon garlic powder
• 1 Teaspoon paprika

- 1 Teaspoon oregano
- 1 bay leaf
- 1 yellow or red potato, chopped

Instructions

1. In a large soup pot, over medium-high heat, brown ground beef.

2. Add frozen vegetables, barley, broth, tomatoes, garlic powder, paprika, oregano and bay leaf. Bring the pot to a boil, Reduce heat, cover and simmer for 15 minutes.

3. Add the potatoes and allow to simmer again for another 20 minutes or until they are tender.

Couscous with Vegetables

- Cuisine Pasta
- Course Main Dishes
- Serves: 4

Ingredients

- 1 1/2 Cup chicken broth

- 1 Cup couscous

- 4 Tablespoons olive oil, divided

- red onion, chopped

- garlic cloves, minced

- tomatoes, seeded, chopped

- yellow bell pepper, seeded and chopped

- red bell pepper, seeded and chopped

- zucchinis, seeded, chopped

- 1 Cup peas, thawed from frozen

- 2 Tablespoons balsamic vinegar

- 2 Tablespoons Feta cheese, crumbled

Instructions

1. In a medium saucepan, over high heat, bring chicken broth and 1 tbs of olive oil to a boil. Remove from heat and stir in couscous. Cover and let sit for 5-10 minutes.

2. In a separate pan over medium heat, add the remaining oil and cook the onions and garlic until softened.

3. Mix in the tomatoes, bell peppers and zucchinis. Cook and stir until tender.

4. Add peas and cook 2-3 more minutes. Add vinegar and cheese and toss to combine.

5. Spoon vegetable mixture over couscous. Serve.

Spinach and Ham Pizza

- Course Main Dishes
- Serves: 4
- Prep time: 15m
- Cook Time: 12m

Ingredients

- 1 store bought baked thin crust whole wheat pizza shell
- 4 Cups baby spinach leaves, sliced thinly
- 1/2 Cup Mushrooms
- 2 Tablespoons olive oil
- 3 Ounces ham or prosciutto
- 1/4 Cup feta cheese, crumbled
- 1/4 Cup Parmesan cheese, grated
- 3 Pieces garlic cloves, sliced thinly

Instructions

1. Preheat oven to 450F degrees.

2. Place the pizza shell on a cookie sheet. Scatter spinach and mushrooms all over crust. Drizzle with oil. Place ham or prosciutto, cheeses, and garlic on top of spinach & mushroom.

3. Bake for 10-12 minutes, until crust is golden brown and spinach is wilted.

Chapter 11: Diverticulitis Smoothie Recipes

Banana Breakfast Smoothie

- Course Breakfast
- Serves: 1 Smoothie

Ingredients

- 1 medium banana
- 1 Cup milk, almond or regular
- 1/2 Cup plain yogurt
- 1/4 Cup 100% Bran flakes
- 1 Teaspoon vanilla extract
- 2 Teaspoons honey or agave syrup
- 1/2 Cup ice
- 1 Pinch cinnamon
- 1 Pinch nutmeg

Instructions

1. Combine all ingredients in a blender and process on medium speed until smooth.

2. Garnish with cinnamon and/or nutmeg.

Tropical Fruit Smoothie

• Course: Breakfast

• Serves: 2

Ingredients

• 1 Cup mix of mangoes, pineapples, bananas

• 1 Cup plain or vanilla yogurt

• 1/2 Cup All Bran cereal

• 1 Teaspoon vanilla

• 1 Tablespoon honey, or agave nectar, optional

• 1 Cup almond or coconut milk or water

• 1/2 avocado

• 1 Cup ice

Instructions

1. Combine all ingredients in a blender and process on high speed until smooth and creamy.

ANTI-INFLAMMATORY BLUEBERRY SMOOTHIE

PREP TIME: 5 minutes

TOTAL TIME: 5 minutes

SERVINGS: 1

INGREDIENTS

- 1 cup almond milk
- 1 frozen banana
- 2/3 – 1 cup frozen blueberries
- 2 handfuls spinach or leafy greens
- 1 T almond butter
- 1/4 tsp cinnamon
- 1/8 – 1/4 tsp cayenne, start light and add as desired
- 1 tsp maca powder, optional

INSTRUCTIONS

- Combine all ingredients in a high powered blender and blend until smooth. Serve immediately.

Healing Green Smoothie

Course: Drinks

Prep Time: 10 minutes

Total Time: 10 minutes

Servings: 6

Calories: 69kcal

Ingredients

• 4-5 large leaves of romaine lettuce

• 3 larges leaves of kale

• 1 large Granny Smith apple cut into slices with seeds removed

• 3 cups of water

• 1 cup of chopped carrots

• 6 medium strawberries

• 1-2 celery stalks

• ½ avocado peeled and pit removed

Instructions

• Place lettuce leaves, kale leaves, and Granny Smith apple slices in Vitamix (or blender).4-5 large leaves of romaine lettuce, 3 larges leaves of kale, 1 large Granny Smith apple

• Add three cups of water.

• Chop up one cup of carrots and add to Vitamix.1 cup of chopped carrots

• Next add strawberries, celery stalks, and avocado.6 medium strawberries, 1-2 celery stalks, ½ avocado

• Blend on smoothie setting.

• Pour into glasses and enjoy.

Pineapple Green Smoothie

Course: Beverage

Cuisine: Smoothie

Prep Time: 5 minutes

Total Time: 5 minutes

Servings: 2

Calories: 131kcal

Equipment

• High speed blender

Ingredients

• 1 cup non-dairy milk, (I used unsweetened coconut milk beverage)

• 1 frozen banana

• 1 cup baby spinach

• 1 cup pineapple chunks, (fresh or frozen)

Instructions

• Blend all the ingredients in a high-speed blender, such as a Vitamix. Enjoy.

Blueberry Gut Healing Protein Shake

Prep: 5 mins

Total: 5 mins

Yield: 2 shakes

Ingredients:

• ¼-1/2 cup of organic frozen blueberries

• 1 cup of organic full-fat coconut milk in the can

• 2 scoops of Gut Healing Protein or another protein powder of your choice that is good for healing the gut (the nutrition info is based on the Gut Healing protein though!)

• 1 tsp of organic cinnamon

Optional Ingredients:

• 1 scoop of organic greens powder. I use Organic Supergreens

Instructions:

1. Gather ingredients

2. Take the coconut milk out of the can (it is often divided into a clumpy, fat portion and water portion) and put it into a blender and blend until smooth and creamy. I will often blend up 2 cans at a time and then place the whipped up coconut milk into a glass mason jar.

3. Add in the frozen organic blueberries, gut healing protein, cinnamon and greens (if you desire).

4. Serve and enjoy.

Brazilian Health Smoothie – Brazilian Root and Fruit

Course: Smoothies

Cuisine: Brazilian

Prep Time: 15 minutes

Servings: 1 servings

Equipment

• Blender or food processor

• Cutting board and knife

• Box Grater

Ingredients

• 1/2 cup Grated raw beets

• 1/2 cup Grated raw carrots

• 1/2 Ripe banana

• 3 Strawberries

• 1/4 tsp Raw ginger root

• 1 tsp Honey

• 1 tbsp Protein powder

• 1/2 cup Water

• 1/4 cup Ice

Instructions

• Place the grated carrots, beets and chopped ginger root into the blender. Pour a little water into the blender and pulse a few times to breakdown the vegetables.

• Cut up the banana half and add to the blender along with the chopped strawberries, protein powder, remaining water, ice and honey and puree to a creamy smoothie.

Gut Soothing Smoothie

PREP TIME: 5 minutes

EQUIPMENT

• Blender

INGREDIENTS

• 1/2 cup canned pumpkin

• 1 banana frozen will make this smoothie creamier and thicker

• 1/2 cup almond milk, more or less for desired thickness no additives or gums

• 1 scoop collagen or bone broth protein

INSTRUCTIONS

• Add everything to blender and blend.

NutriBullet Heart-Healthy Hemp Smoothie Recipe

Yield: 1

Prep time: 2 MINUTES

Cook time: 1 MINUTE

Total time: 3 MINUTES

Ingredients

• 1/4 avocado

• 1 clementine, peeled

• 1 date, pitted

• 1 cup mixed berries, frozen

• 1 cup hemp milk, unsweetened

• 1 tbsp cacao powder

• 1 tbsp hemp seeds

• 1/2 cup water

• 1 scoop Collagen Boost, optional

Instructions

1. Place avocado, clementine, dates, mixed berries, hemp milk, water, cacao nibs, and hemp seeds into a NutriBullet blender and secure the lid.

2. Start the blender on its lowest speed and steadily ramp up to its highest speed. This will reduce wear and tear on the motor and blades, facilitate a more consistent blend, and help prevent food splatter onto the lid and sides.

3. Blend for approximately 30 seconds or until a smooth consistency is achieved.

4. Pour into a glass for immediate refreshment or place in the refrigerator in an airtight container to enjoy later.

Notes

1. If you don't have frozen fruit, or simply prefer to use fresh fruit (we totally get that), we recommend adding 1/2 cup of ice to chill your smoothie and give it a pleasing icy texture.

2. Almond milk or coconut milk can be substituted for the hemp milk and still keep this delicious smoothie dairy-free.

3. Oranges can be substituted for the clementines without significantly changing the flavor profile.

Detoxifying Super Green Smoothie

- Total Time: 6 minutes
- Yield: 2

Ingredients

- 2 kiwis, peeled
- 1 lime juiced
- 1 lemon, juiced
- 6 ounces fresh celery juice (5-6 large celery stalks) or unsweetened coconut water
- 4 ounces fresh squeezed orange juice
- 1 sprig parsley
- ½ teaspoon ground ginger
- Pinch kosher salt
- Optional- small handful baby spinach (slightly steam and cool before adding to blender, for better digestion), 1 Tablespoon chia seeds or 2 Tablespoons vegan protein powder, 1 teaspoon maple syrup or honey

Instructions

1. Place all ingredients in a blender and blend until combined. Add ice to the blender if, desired, or serve over ice.

2. Serve and enjoy immediately.

Notes

1. Add vegan protein powder chia seeds to boost the protein in this smoothie.

Creamy Pineapple Cucumber Smoothie

PREP TIME: 5 minutes

TOTAL TIME: 5 minutes

Ingredients

• 1/2 cup sliced cucumber (skin on / organic when possible)

• 1 heaping cup cubed pineapple (if frozen, omit ice)

• 1/2 large ripe, peeled, frozen banana

• 1/4 cup light coconut milk

• 1/2 cup filtered water

• 1 medium lime, zested + juiced (1 tsp zest / 2 Tbsp (30 ml) juice per 1 lime)

- 1 large handful greens (spinach or kale / organic when possible)
- 2-4 ice cubes

Instructions

- Add cucumber, pineapple, frozen banana, light coconut milk, water, lime zest, lime juice, greens, and ice cubes to a blender and blend on high until creamy and smooth, scraping down sides as needed.
- For a thicker smoothie, add more ice. For a thinner smoothie, add more liquid of choice. Taste and adjust flavor as needed, adding more lime juice or zest for acidity/brightness, banana or pineapple for sweetness, coconut milk for creaminess, and greens for more intense green color.
- Serve immediately. Leftovers will keep covered in the refrigerator up to 24 hours, though best when fresh.

Low Oxalate Smoothie

Prep Time: 5 minutes

Cook Time: 0 minutes

Total Time: 5 minutes

Ingredients

- 1/2 banana
- 1/2 cup frozen cherries (or other low oxalate fruit)
- 1 tablespoon flaxseed
- 1/2 cup 2% milk (or plain kefir)
- 1/4 cup lowfat plain yogurt

Instructions

- Combine all ingredients in a blender.
- Blend until smooth.
- Enjoy.

BANANA NUTMEG SMOOTHIE

Ready In: 5mins

Ingredients: 4

Serves: 2

INGREDIENTS

- 1 banana
- 1 1/2 cups milk (or soy milk)
- 1 tablespoon honey
- 1/4 teaspoon freshly grated nutmeg

DIRECTIONS

1. Combine all the ingredients in a blender and process until smooth.

Chapter 12: 30 Days Meal Plan for Diverticulitis Diet

Week 1:

Day 1:

1. Breakfast: Oatmeal with bananas and honey

2. Lunch: Chicken and vegetable soup

3. Dinner: Baked salmon with steamed broccoli

4. Snack: Greek yogurt with berries

Day 2:

1. Breakfast: Smoothie (spinach, banana, almond milk)

2. Lunch: Turkey and avocado wrap

3. Dinner: Lentil soup with carrots and celery

4. Snack: Applesauce with cinnamon

Day 3:

1. Breakfast: Greek yogurt with honey and soft fruit

2. Lunch: Quinoa salad with cucumbers and tomatoes

3. Dinner: Grilled chicken with sweet potato

4. Snack: Smoothie (mango, coconut milk)

Day 4:

1. Breakfast: Mango smoothie

2. Lunch: Vegetable broth with soft vegetables

3. Dinner: Baked cod with zucchini

4. Snack: Soft cheese and whole grain crackers

Day 5:

1. Breakfast: Soft-boiled eggs and whole-grain toast

2. Lunch: Mixed greens salad with light dressing

3. Dinner: Turkey meatballs with brown rice

4. Snack: Hummus with cucumber slices

Day 6:

1. Breakfast: Banana and almond butter on whole-grain toast

2. Lunch: Vegetable stir-fry (carrots, zucchini, bell peppers)

3. Dinner: Chicken breast with mashed potatoes

4. Snack: Smoothie (berries, lactose-free yogurt)

Day 7:

1. Breakfast: Oatmeal with honey and soft fruit

2. Lunch: Lentil and vegetable stew

3. Dinner: Grilled tilapia with quinoa

4. Snack: Rice pudding

Week 2:

Day 8:

1. Breakfast: Smoothie (blueberries, spinach, almond milk)

2. Lunch: Soft cheese and turkey wrap

3. Dinner: Baked chicken with steamed carrots

4. Snack: Chia seed pudding

Day 9:

1. Breakfast: Greek yogurt with honey and berries

2. Lunch: Chicken and avocado salad

3. Dinner: Baked salmon with quinoa

4. Snack: Applesauce with cinnamon

Day 10:

1. Breakfast: Oatmeal with bananas

2. Lunch: Lentil soup with spinach

3. Dinner: Grilled chicken with steamed broccoli

4. Snack: Smoothie (mango, coconut milk)

Day 11:

1. Breakfast: Soft-boiled eggs and whole-grain toast

2. Lunch: Mixed greens salad with light dressing

3. Dinner: Turkey meatballs with brown rice

4. Snack: Hummus with carrot sticks

Day 12:

1. Breakfast: Banana and almond butter on whole-grain toast

2. Lunch: Vegetable stir-fry (carrots, zucchini, bell peppers)

3. Dinner: Chicken breast with mashed potatoes

4. Snack: Greek yogurt with honey

Day 13:

1. Breakfast: Smoothie (spinach, banana, almond milk)

2. Lunch: Quinoa salad with cucumbers and tomatoes

3. Dinner: Baked cod with zucchini

4. Snack: Soft cheese and whole grain crackers

Day 14:

1. Breakfast: Greek yogurt with berries

2. Lunch: Chicken and vegetable soup

3. Dinner: Baked salmon with steamed broccoli

4. Snack: Applesauce with cinnamon

Week 3:

Day 15:

1. Breakfast: Smoothie (blueberries, spinach, almond milk)

2. Lunch: Soft cheese and turkey wrap

3. Dinner: Baked chicken with steamed carrots

4. Snack: Chia seed pudding

Day 16:

1. Breakfast: Oatmeal with bananas and honey

2. Lunch: Chicken and avocado salad

3. Dinner: Baked salmon with quinoa

4. Snack: Smoothie (mango, coconut milk)

Day 17:

1. Breakfast: Greek yogurt with honey and berries

2. Lunch: Lentil soup with carrots and celery

3. Dinner: Grilled chicken with sweet potato

4. Snack: Applesauce with cinnamon

Day 18:

1. Breakfast: Soft-boiled eggs and whole-grain toast

2. Lunch: Mixed greens salad with light dressing

3. Dinner: Turkey meatballs with brown rice

4. Snack: Hummus with cucumber slices

Day 19:

1. Breakfast: Banana and almond butter on whole-grain toast

2. Lunch: Vegetable stir-fry (carrots, zucchini, bell peppers)

3. Dinner: Chicken breast with mashed potatoes

4. Snack: Smoothie (berries, lactose-free yogurt)

Day 20:

1. Breakfast: Oatmeal with honey and soft fruit

2. Lunch: Quinoa salad with cucumbers and tomatoes

3. Dinner: Baked cod with zucchini

4. Snack: Greek yogurt with honey

Day 21:

1. Breakfast: Smoothie (spinach, banana, almond milk)

2. Lunch: Chicken and vegetable soup

3. Dinner: Grilled tilapia with quinoa

4. Snack: Rice pudding

Week 4:

Day 22:

1. Breakfast: Greek yogurt with honey and berries

2. Lunch: Lentil and vegetable stew

3. Dinner: Baked salmon with steamed broccoli

4. Snack: Applesauce with cinnamon

Day 23:

1. Breakfast: Oatmeal with bananas

2. Lunch: Chicken and avocado salad

3. Dinner: Baked salmon with quinoa

4. Snack: Smoothie (mango, coconut milk)

Day 24:

1. Breakfast: Soft-boiled eggs and whole-grain toast

2. Lunch: Mixed greens salad with light dressing

3. Dinner: Turkey meatballs with brown rice

4. Snack: Hummus with carrot sticks

Day 25:

1. Breakfast: Smoothie (spinach, banana, almond milk)

2. Lunch: Quinoa salad with cucumbers and tomatoes

3. Dinner: Baked cod with zucchini

4. Snack: Soft cheese and whole grain crackers

Day 26:

1. Breakfast: Greek yogurt with honey and berries

2. Lunch: Chicken and vegetable soup

3. Dinner: Grilled chicken with sweet potato

4. Snack: Applesauce with cinnamon

Day 27:

1. Breakfast: Oatmeal with honey and soft fruit

2. Lunch: Lentil soup with spinach

3. Dinner: Baked salmon with quinoa

4. Snack: Smoothie (mango, coconut milk)

Day 28:

1. Breakfast: Banana and almond butter on whole-grain toast

2. Lunch: Vegetable stir-fry (carrots, zucchini, bell peppers)

3. Dinner: Chicken breast with mashed potatoes

4. Snack: Greek yogurt with honey

Day 29:

1. Breakfast: Smoothie (blueberries, spinach, almond milk)

2. Lunch: Soft cheese and turkey wrap

3. Dinner: Baked chicken with steamed carrots

4. Snack: Chia seed pudding

Day 30:

1. Breakfast: Greek yogurt with berries

2. Lunch: Chicken and avocado salad

3. Dinner: Grilled tilapia with quinoa

4. Snack: Rice pudding

CONCLUSION

Navigating the complexities of a diverticulitis diet involves more than just choosing the right foods; it requires a holistic approach to nutrition, hydration, and meal planning. A diverticulitis-friendly diet prioritizes gentle, easily digestible foods that minimize irritation while providing essential nutrients. By incorporating a variety of proteins, soft vegetables, and hydrating beverages, individuals can manage their symptoms effectively and maintain overall health.

Personalization is key-what works for one person may not work for another. This is why a flexible, customizable meal plan is crucial. Listening to your body and making adjustments based on your unique responses can significantly enhance your comfort and well-being.

Moreover, the importance of preparation and mindful eating cannot be overstated. Taking time to plan meals, batch cook, and store foods properly can reduce stress and ensure you have safe, nourishing options readily available.

Simple strategies like creating shopping lists, investing in quality storage containers, and dedicating a day to meal prep can make a world of difference.

Ultimately, managing diverticulitis through diet is a journey of trial and error, patience, and continuous learning. By embracing a balanced, nutrient-rich approach, you can not only alleviate symptoms but also foster a healthier, more enjoyable relationship with food. This journey is about more than just managing a condition-it's about reclaiming your quality of life and savoring the simple pleasures of eating well.

www.ingramcontent.com/pod-product-compliance
Lightning Source LLC
Chambersburg PA
CBHW061046250726
48653CB00001B/281